Co

and Hypertension

Michael Schachter

Senior Lecturer
Department of Clinical Pharmacology and Therapeutics
National Heart and Lung Institute
Faculty of Medicine
Imperial College
St Mary's Hospital
London, UK

MARTIN DUNITZ

Although every effort has been made to ensure that drug doses and other information are presented accurately in this publication, the ultimate responsibility rests with the prescribing physician. Neither the publishers nor the authors can be held responsible for errors or for any consequences arising from the use of information contained herein. Any product mentioned in this publication should be used in accordance with the prescribing information prepared by the manufacturers. No claims or endorsements are made for any drug or compound at present under clinical investigation.

The views expressed in this publication are those of the author and not necessarily those of Martin Dunitz Ltd.

First published in the United Kingdom in 2002 by
Martin Dunitz Ltd
The Livery House
7–9 Pratt Street, London NW1 0AE

Tel: +44 (0)207 482 2202
Fax: +44 (0)207 267 0159
E-mail: info.dunitz@tandf.co.uk
Website: http://www.dunitz.co.uk

A CIP record for this book is available from the British Library

ISBN 1–85317–732–6

Distributed in the USA by:
Fulfilment Center, Taylor & Francis, 7625 Empire Drive, Florence, KY 41042, USA
Toll free Tel: +1 800 634 7064 E-mail: cserve@routledge_ny.com

Distributed in Canada by:
Taylor & Francis, 74 Rolark Drive, Scarborough, Ontario, M1R 4G2, Canada
Toll free Tel: +1 877 226 2237 E-mail: tal_fran@istar.ca

Distributed in the rest of the world by:
ITPS Limited, Cheriton House, North Way, Andover, Hampshire, SP10 5BE, UK
Tel: +44 (0) 1264 332424 E-mail: reception@itps.co.uk

Printed and bound in Italy by Printer Trento S.r.l.

Contents

Preface

Interest in hypertension and its management shows no signs of abating. In the past 2–3 years there has been a flood of guidelines on this subject from national and international organizations. How far this affects management is another matter, in a profession already suffering from guideline fatigue. Some points are, however, generally accepted by everyone involved in treating hypertension and other cardiovascular problems: hypertension is common; it is relatively under-treated throughout the world; and in order to improve this situation most patients will need treatment with two or more drugs. This short book deals with current ideas on such combination therapy and the evidence available (and missing). I hope it will prove of some use in guiding readers through this increasingly complex field. But it certainly is not intended as a comprehensive textbook on the management of hypertension. Even with this exclusion it goes without saying that the literature on these topics is enormous and constantly expanding. Rather than interrupt the text constantly with references I have chosen to group all 'further reading' together at the end of the book, mostly under the individual chapter headings with some general references also included.

The problem of hypertension

The epidemiology of hypertension – who and where

This heading is obviously inadequate in an important respect: how do we actually define hypertension? The question is not as straightforward as it might seem, nor is the answer to the question constant. There has been a consistent lowering of the level of blood pressure that is considered 'hypertension'. This will be discussed in more detail later in this book, in the context of treatment targets. However, it is clearly important to have an overview of the size of the problem. More than 20 different criteria have been described and clearly they will produce widely differing results. The US Third National Health and Nutrition Examination Survey (NHANES III) is a useful starting point, defining hypertension as a systolic blood pressure (SBP) equal to or greater than 140 mmHg, a diastolic blood pressure (DBP) of 90 mmHg or more, or simply being on antihypertensive medication. On this basis, about 20% of the adult population of the USA was considered to be hypertensive. This overall figure actually conceals a number of significant differences:

- The prevalence of hypertension rises steadily with *age*, at least in Westernized societies. This is largely due to the progressive increase in SBP combined with those who had developed combined systolic and diastolic hypertension in middle age. In patients over the age of 65, isolated systolic hypertension (ISH) is usually the dominant form of hypertension. Over the age of 70 the prevalence of ISH, defined as SBP ≥ 140 mmHg and DBP < 90 mmHg, may be two in three of the population.

- There are marked differences in the prevalence of hypertension in different *ethnic groups*. Hypertension is much more frequent in black Americans than in white Americans, and this is also true of the situation in the UK. In addition, blacks seem to be at greater risk than whites of some types of target organ damage such as left ventricular hypertrophy. There appears to be a strong genetic link which extends to the West African populations from which the majority of these patients originate. At the same time it has been shown that East Africans in rural communities have a low prevalence of hypertension, which rises sharply on migration to the cities. In general, the prevalence of hypertension in whites in industrialized countries is similar to that in the USA.

Notwithstanding these differences, there is no dispute that hypertension is a very substantial problem for clinical medicine and public health, and one that is likely to increase in the many countries in which the average age of the population is also increasing. It is worth noting that there have been historic discrepancies in the complications of hypertension in different populations — for instance, coronary disease has been comparatively rare despite the high prevalence of hypertension, while stroke has been common — but this situation is now changing. The visible consequence is increased coronary artery disease in Japan and in other countries in which it was previously uncommon. The most obvious cause is the 'Westernization' of diet, with increased use of saturated fats, but this explanation may be far too simplistic.

Secondary hypertension

This book is concerned with primary or 'essential' hypertension and its management. However, secondary hypertension should

Table 1 *Causes of secondary hypertension.*

Increased renin secretion
Renovascular disease
Renin-secreting tumours (*very rare*)
Increased adrenocortical hormones
Primary hyperaldosteronism (Conn's syndrome)
Deoxycorticosterone excess (11beta-hydroxylase deficiency)
Corticosteroid excess (Cushing's syndrome, primary or secondary)
Increased catecholamines
Phaeochromocytoma
Secondary to drugs, etc
Steroids
Liquorice (in large quantities!), carbenoxolone
Sympathomimetics
Other causes
Pregnancy-related hypertension (including pre-eclampsia)
Coarctation of the aorta

be mentioned briefly. Overall, the various types combined account for no more than 15% of cases of hypertension, and probably nearer 5% in the middle-aged population. Causes are listed in Table 1.

Causes of 'essential' hypertension – theories and controversies

Perhaps fortunately, this book has neither the space nor the intention of dealing with this subject in detail. The cause or causes of so-called essential hypertension has prompted a vast body of research and great controversy, some of it more sectarian than rational. Since the issue remains unresolved, and is not in any case likely to have a simple solution, it is perhaps not surprising that our treatment of this disorder is far from perfect: indeed, it may more be surprising that it is not worse. The main lines of thought and research can be summarized as follows:

- Hypertension is primarily a disorder of the *central nervous system* and specifically of *sympathetic dysregulation and hyperactivity*. A variant of this theory suggests that there is correctable vascular compression of the rostral ventrolateral medulla, a part of the brain stem crucially involved in the up-regulation of sympathetic outflow.
- Hypertension is the result of interaction between *environmental factors*, notably *high salt intake* and *psychosocial stress*, and the individual's genetic predisposition to hypertension. The sympathetic nervous system may then be the effector pathway for increase in blood pressure.
- Hypertension is primarily a *renal disorder*, specifically associated with *abnormal sodium handling*. Clearly, this may be related to the second hypothesis above. Some hypertensives, particularly with relatively young onset, have high renin concentrations for unknown reasons.
- Underlying any or all of these hypotheses, as already indicated, is the question of *genetic predisposition*. This question is currently the subject of intensive research, though it is extremely improbable that a single gene will be the underlying cause of essential hypertension. So far the identified genetic contribution accounts for much less than half the variability of blood pressure.
- It is widely believed that, in a substantial minority of patients, hypertension forms part of a *metabolic syndrome arising from insulin resistance* (Figure 1) — that is to say, inadequate glucose uptake in response to high concentrations of insulin, particularly in skeletal muscle. Characteristically, these patients are middle-aged men with central obesity, non-insulin

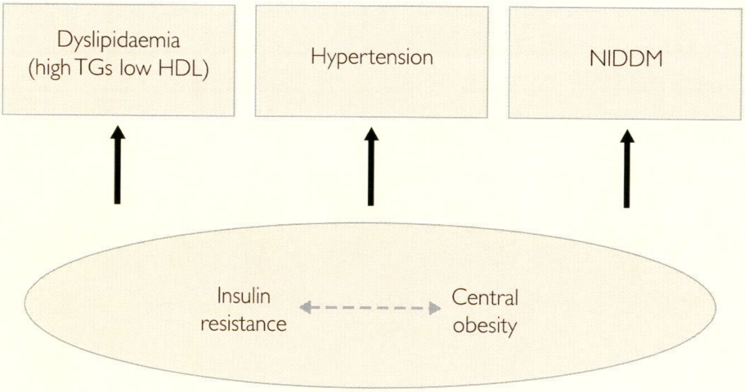

HDL: high-density lipoproteins; NIDDM: non-insulin dependent diabetes mellitus; TG: triglyceride.

Figure 1 *Metabolic syndrome arising from insulin resistance.*

dependent diabetes or at least impaired glucose tolerance, and dyslipidaemia, in addition to hypertension.

- Hypertension is characterized by changes in *vascular structure and function* throughout the circulation, particularly in the microvasculature. Overall, there is an increase in peripheral resistance which may be due to (a) reduced lumen size in resistance arteries and arterioles (Figure 2) or (b) reduction in the number of small vessels (especially capillaries), a process known as rarefaction. It must be remembered that:

  blood pressure = peripheral resistance × cardiac output

  but also that ISH represents a special case, which will be discussed later.

- It is a universally accepted basis of clinical practice that treatment should be based on understanding of the causes of disease. Hypertension is far from unique in that currently we can only aspire to this understanding, although we do have a reasonable comprehension of the pathophysiological mechanisms. Whether this understanding is actually helpful in practice is an interesting issue, which will be discussed later.

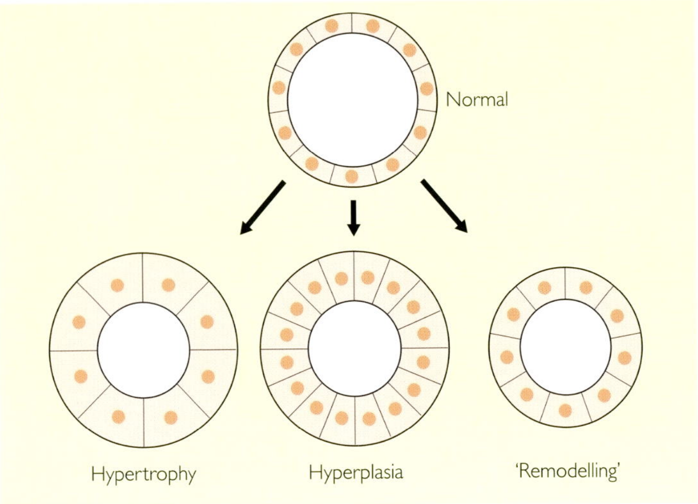

Figure 2 *Hypertensive changes in vascular structure and function: reduced lumen size in resistance arteries and arterioles.*

Hypertension and total cardiovascular risk

Sir George Pickering, one of the pioneers of hypertension research in the UK, commented that the trouble with doctors was that they could only count to two. He meant by this that clinicians are used to situations in which the patient either does or does not have a disorder, like pneumonia or bronchial carcinoma.

Hypertension is different. The doctor is making a judgment about a continuous variable. Is an SBP of 161 mmHg really hypertensive, while one of 159 mmHg entirely normal? So often, the answer is : 'it depends'. It is now appreciated that hypertension needs to be seen in the context of the patient's overall cardiovascular risk. Major epidemiological studies, notably at Framingham in New England but also in Munster in Germany and elsewhere, have provided estimates of this risk, and there are charts and formulae based on these data that incorporate information on total and high-density lipoprotein (HDL) cholesterol, smoking, and diabetes, as well as blood pressure. For instance, the British Hypertension Society guidelines include a Framingham-derived chart for the calculation of risk in terms of cardiovascular events per 5 or 10 years. One can therefore set a threshold for intervention based on, say, a 10-year risk of 20% or 30%. This method is certainly appropriate, both in principle and practice, in making decisions about treatment, but it does not really avoid the 'binary' problem. Is a 19% risk acceptable and a 21% risk the grounds for one or more interventions? Ultimately — reassuringly perhaps — there must remain scope for the clinician's judgment. Table 2 summarizes recent guidelines from

Table 2 *Some key points from recently published hypertension guidelines.*

US Joint National Committee, 6th report, 1997
General target blood pressure <140/90 mmHg
Same target in elderly; interim target systolic pressure of <160 mmHg in ISH
Target pressure for diabetic patients should be <130/85 mmHg
Diuretics and beta-blockers considered initially, but consider other factors that may favour alternative drugs (see Table 8)
World Health Organization/International Society of Hypertension, 1999
General target blood pressure <130/85 mmHg
Similar for diabetic patients
Target <140/90 mmHg in the elderly
Choice of drug dependent on patient's clinical context
British Hypertension Society, 1999
Target blood pressure <140/85 mmHg
Acceptable level for audit <150/90 mmHg
Similar targets for the elderly
Target in diabetes <140/80 mmHg but <130/80 mmHg in presence of proteinuria
Thiazide usual first-choice drug but consider context (see Table 8)

* ISH: isolated systolic hypertension.

major organizations while Table 3 shows risk categories as defined by the World Health Organization and International Society of Hypertension.

Table 3 *Categories of risk in hypertension as defined by WHO/ISH guidelines.*

	Grade I (mild hypertension) SBP 140-159 or DBP 90-99	Grade II (moderate) SBP 160-179 or DBP 100-109	Grade III (severe) SBP ≥ 180 or DBP ≥ 110
No other risk factors	Low	Med	High
1-2 risk factors*	Med	Med	Very high
3 or more risk factors or target organ damage or diabetes	High	High	Very high
Associated clinical conditions†	Very high	Very high	Very high

DBP: diastolic blood pressure; SBP: systolic blood pressure.
* Men >55 years, women >65 years, smoking, diabetes, positive family history, raised cholesterol; †eg, history of stroke, heart failure, renal disease, peripheral vascular disease.

The treatment of hypertension

Hypertension is a chronic, indeed usually a life-long, disorder. It is therefore understandable that many people will seek alternatives to years or even decades of drug treatment. The list of potential non-pharmacological therapies is correspondingly a long one. They are described in Table 4, with some comments. Although several of these interventions are desirable and well-founded in terms of clinical evidence, it is only realistic to recognize that many patients will not adhere to them and that their efficacy is limited. In fact, most patients will require drug therapy.

Table 4 *Non-pharmacological treatments in hypertension.*

Weight loss	
Reduced salt intake*	
Reduced alcohol consumption†	
Exercise (aerobic)	
Potassium supplementation*	
Calcium supplementation*	
Magnesium supplementation*	
Stress management	– relaxation therapy – meditation – yoga

*Several combinations reported; †in individuals with high initial intakes – may be closely related to weight.

Available drug therapies — advantages and disadvantages

Compared with 20, or even 5, years ago, today's prescriber has a huge choice of antihypertensive agents. This does not make his or her decisions any easier, particularly since views on specific drug classes can change quickly. Table 5 summarizes the major classes of existing drugs.

Diuretics (especially thiazides)

Mechanism of action

Although thiazide diuretics are among the longest-established and probably the most extensively tested antihypertensive drugs, we still have a very poor understanding of their mechanism of action. As might be expected, they produce both volume depletion and sodium loss at first, accompanied by a fall in peripheral resistance (sometimes briefly preceded by an increase) and cardiac output. With chronic use (more than a couple of months) lowered peripheral resistance and increased sodium excretion persist, but cardiac output and blood volume gradually return to pre-treatment levels (Figure 3). A direct vasodilator effect may be relevant at this stage but has proved difficult to demonstrate.

Advantages

- Very good evidence of efficacy and long-term reduction in stroke and cardiovascular events, especially in the elderly.
- Very low cost.
- Convenient dosage regime.

Disadvantages

- Potential metabolic abnormalities — hypokalaemia and hyponatraemia, hyperuricaemia, impaired glucose tolerance, worsening lipid profile, hypomagnesaemia (these can be minimized by low

Table 5 *Antihypertensive drugs available in the UK (early 2000).*

1. 'First-line drugs'

Diuretics
- *Thiazides*
- *Potassium-sparing*

Beta-blockers
- *Without vasodilator activity*
- *With vasodilator activity*
  - with $alpha_1$-blocking properties
  - with intrinsic agonist activity
  - with other vasodilator activity

Calcium channel blockers
- *Dihydropyridines*
- *Others*
  - Verapamil
  - Diltiazem

Angiotensin converting enzyme inhibitors and receptor antagonists
- *Angiotensin converting enzyme inhibitors*
- *Angiotensin receptor antagonists (AT_1 antagonists)*

$Alpha_1$-blockers

2. Other antihypertensive drugs ('alternative first line')

Centrally acting drugs
- Reserpine
- Methyldopa
- Clonidine
- Moxonidine

Adrenergic neurone blockers (*largely obsolete*)

Vasodilators with various mechanisms of action
- Diazoxide
- Hydrallazine
- Minoxidil
- Sodium nitroprusside (IV only)

doses, and hypokalaemia specifically by concurrent potassium-sparing diuretics such as amiloride, or ACE inhibitors).

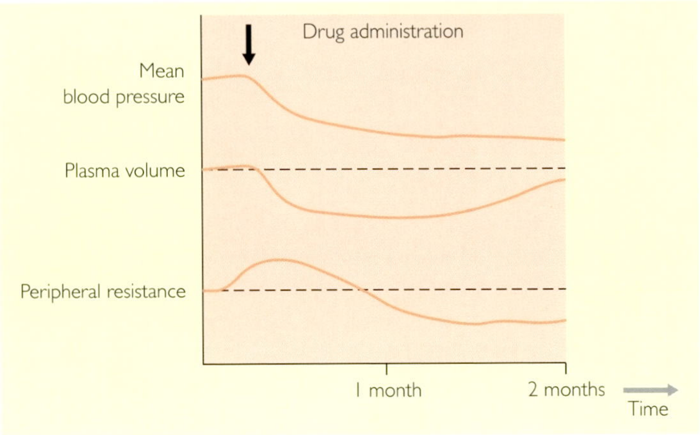

Figure 3 *Thiazide diuretics: mechanism of action.*

- May cause postural hypotension.
- May cause impotence.
- Rare liver, bone marrow and skin toxicity.

Beta-blockers

Mechanism of action

Once again, the exact mechanism of action of these very well-established drugs is uncertain, but the general view is that lowering of blood pressure is associated with diminished cardiac output in the presence of peripheral resistance that may actually increase: 'pure' beta-blockers are not vasodilators (Figure 4). For drugs with partial agonist activity (so-called intrinsic sympathomimetic activity, or ISA) such as pindolol, there may, however some fall in peripheral resistance with a less marked lowering in cardiac output, probably caused at least partly by vasodilatation. Some other beta-blockers have definite vasodilator activity from $alpha_1$-adrenergic blockade (labetalol) or have a direct action on smooth muscle (nebivolol). The eventual outcome is much the same, resulting from a *relative* fall in periph-

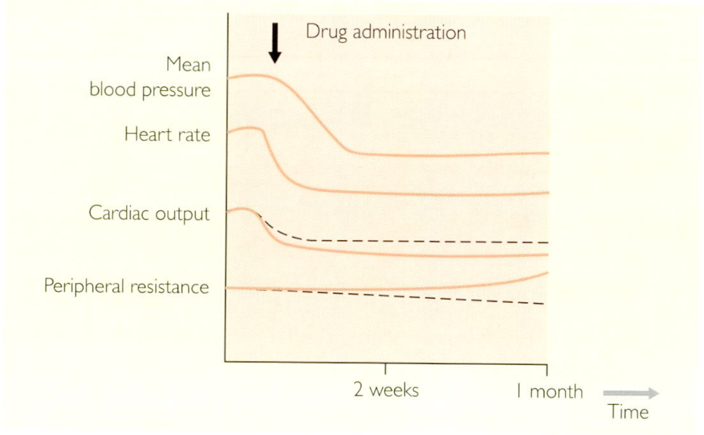

Figure 4 *Beta-blockers: mechanism of action.*

eral resistance, with or without vasodilatation depending on the specific agent. It must also be remembered that beta-blockers also cause a lowering in renin secretion, which can contribute significantly to blood pressure lowering in patients with high-renin hypertension: as noted, such patients are usually relatively young. Contrary to statements in most textbooks, *hypotension can be dangerously abrupt* if such patients are given a beta-blocker.

Advantages

- Long-term efficacy and beneficial effects on morbidity and mortality well-proven in trials.
- Useful in patients with co-existing angina.
- Usually simple once-daily dosing.

Disadvantages

- Can cause sinus bradycardia and precipitate heart block.
- Can precipitate or aggravate heart failure because of inhibitory effect on cardiac contractility (negative inotropy).

- Can cause dangerous bronchospasm in patients with asthma or chronic obstructive pulmonary disease.
- May cause deterioration in peripheral vascular disease — of doubtful relevance in atherosclerosis, but important in Raynaud's phenomenon.
- Can worsen lipid profile and impair insulin sensitivity (less marked in drugs with ISA, alpha-blocking or other vasodilator properties).
- May decrease awareness of hypoglycaemia in diabetics (again of dubious clinical importance).
- Can cause sleep disturbance, including nightmares.

Calcium channel blockers

Mechanism of action

This is a large and heterogeneous group of drugs with differing properties, as shown in Table 6. As far as their hypotensive effect is concerned, however, it is likely to be the vasodilator effect which is crucial, with inhibition of calcium entry into blood vessels leading to reduced smooth muscle tone and therefore reduced peripheral resistance.

Advantages

- Short-term efficacy good (note that there are no long-term data on clinical outcome except for the dihydropyridine nitrendipine in the elderly).

Table 6 *Properties of different classes of calcium channel blockers.*

	Myocardial contractility	Cardiac conduction	Vasodilation
Dihydropyridines	A, B	A	E
Phenylalkylamines (verapamil)	C	B	D
Bezothiazepines (diltiazem)	B	B	D

Levels of effect — A: little or none; B: reduced; C: depressed; D: enhanced; E: increased.

- May be useful in angina (especially non-dihydropyridines, or dihydropyridines combined with beta-blockers).
- Few absolute contraindications (eg, safe in asthma, peripheral vascular disease).
- Simple dosage regimes, though sometimes only with modified-release preparations.

Disadvantages

- May cause flushing, headache, ankle oedema (especially dihydropyridines).
- May cause reflex sympathetic activation secondary to vasodilatation (especially short-acting dihydropyridines, which should not be used): tachycardia, possible long-term adverse effects on cardiac events and mortality.
- May cause bradycardia, negative inotropy, in case of non-dihydropyridines.
- Rare gum hyperplasia (particularly dihydropyridines).

Angiotensin converting enzyme (ACE) inhibitors and angiotensin receptor antagonists

Mechanisms of action

Angiotensin II can raise blood pressure by several mechanisms, including the potentiation of sympathetic action (Figure 5). It is not surprising, therefore, that inhibition of angiotensin II formation, or antagonism of vascular angiotensin II receptors (specifically the AT_1 subtype), will lower blood pressure when there is high renin activity. It is perhaps more interesting that these drugs are also effective in some patients with normal or low renin levels. One plausible reason is the fact that ACE inhibitors also affect other enzymes, notably kininase, which is involved in the breakdown of vasodilator peptides such as bradykinin and substance P. In theory this should not apply to the receptor antagonists, though recent data suggest that unopposed activation of the AT_2 receptor can lead to increased bradykinin release.

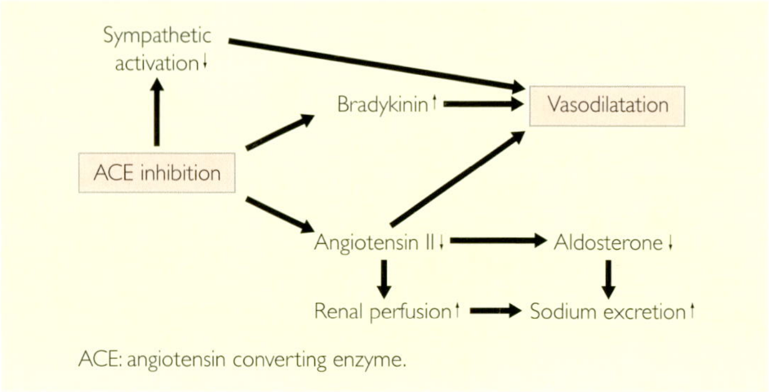

Figure 5 *Mechanisms of action of ACE inhibitors.*

Advantages

- Effective in most patient groups.
- May provide specific renal protection in diabetes.
- Safe in most patients (but see below).
- Long duration of action especially for newer agents (trandolapril, perindopril).
- Enhanced well-being reported in some studies — possible cognitive improvement?
- Receptor antagonists exceptionally well-tolerated.

Disadvantages

- First-dose hypotension, especially in sodium and volume-depleted patients: uncommon with longer-acting agents and the receptor antagonists.
- Irritating cough in 5–20% of patients: much less common with the receptor antagonists.

- May rarely cause anaphylactoid reactions: also very uncommon with the receptor antagonists.
- Deterioration in renal function in patients with renovascular disease, due to altered intrarenal haemodynamics — this can be severe and lead rapidly to renal failure. It is possible that the receptor antagonists can cause similar problems but this has yet to be assessed.

Alpha$_1$-adrenergic blockers

Mechanism of action

The principal mode of action of these drugs is inhibition of noradrenaline-induced vasoconstriction by blocking alpha$_1$-adrenergic receptors in the vascular wall. There may also be some central inhibition of sympathetic activity, though this may be more important in prevention of reflex tachycardia than in lowering blood pressure.

Advantages

- Once-daily dosage for newer compounds.
- Few contraindications.
- Neutral or possibly beneficial metabolic effects, especially on lipid profile: reduced total cholesterol, increased HDL cholesterol.

Disadvantages

- May cause postural hypotension, particularly 'first dose' effect (less likely with new longer-acting agents).
- Can cause tiredness and sedation.
- Dose may need to be titrated over a broad range if used as monotherapy.

Centrally-acting drugs, or sympatholytics

Mechanism of action

All these drugs reduce sympathetic outflow at the level of the brainstem but not all by the same mechanisms (Figure 6). Reserpine, the oldest of these drugs, depletes neurones of norepinephrine and other monoamine neurotransmitters. Methyldopa and clonidine act primarily as agonists at inhibitory pre-synaptic alpha$_2$-adrenergic receptors. The newer drugs moxonidine and rilmenidine are believed to be relatively selective agonists at imidazoline I_1 receptors in the rostral ventrolateral medulla.

Advantages

- Long experience of efficacy, including long-term outcome studies (reserpine).
- Simple dosage.
- Very low cost (reserpine).
- Known to be safe in pregnancy (methyldopa).

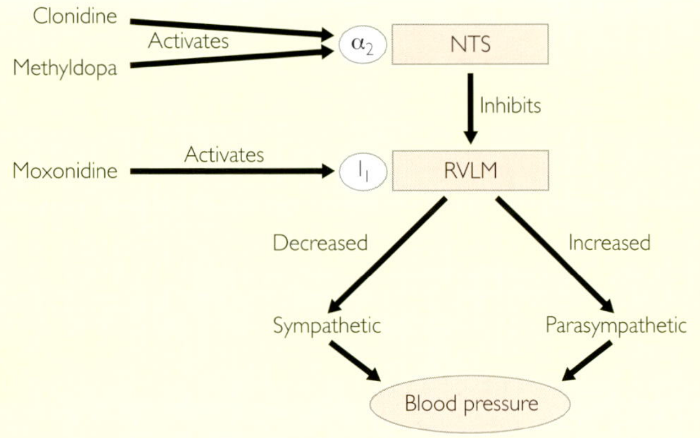

α_2: alpha$_2$ adrenergic receptors; I_1: imidazoline I_1 receptors; NTS: nucleus tractus solitarius; RVLM: rostral ventrolateral medullar.

Figure 6 *Sympatholytics: mechanisms of action.*

- No adverse effects on glucose or lipid metabolism, or in asthma (clonidine, moxonidine especially) — possible improvement in glucose tolerance (moxonidine)?
- Convenient dosage in modified-release form, or transdermal patch (clonidine), or as conventional formulation (moxonidine).

Disadvantages

- Can cause sedation and depression, sometimes severe (reserpine, methyldopa).
- May cause sodium and water retention (less with moxonidine, rilmenidine).
- Dry mouth.
- May cause parkinsonian syndrome (methyldopa).
- Hyperprolactinaemia [galactorrhoea, gynaecomastia] (methyldopa).
- Sometimes causes liver damage, haemolytic anaemia (methyldopa).
- Sexual dysfunction in significant minority of men (not noted with moxonidine, rilmenidine).
- Rebound hypertension (clondine especially — much less likely with modified-release formulations or patches).

The concept of monotherapy

If drug treatment of hypertension were considered necessary, patients and doctors would certainly prefer to use single drug therapy. This is increasingly seen as unrealistic, for reasons that will form the basis of most of the remainder of this book. At this point it is worth noting two US studies, which compared several major classes of antihypertensive agents. The Treatment of Mild Hypertension Study (TOMHS) enrolled more than 900 middle-aged men with DBP between 90 mmHg and 99 mmHg, who were randomly assigned to placebo or one of the following: the beta-blocker acebutolol; the calcium channel blocker amlodipine; the thiazide diuretic chlorthalidone; the alpha-blocker doxazosin; and the ACE inhibitor enalapril. All the treatments were more effective than placebo in lowering systolic and diastolic blood pressure but the differences between them were small, spanning a 3.3 mmHg range for systolic pressure and a 2.5 mmHg range for DBP. After correction for placebo this represented a range from 2.7 mmHg to 6.0 mmHg reduction for SBP and 1.1 mmHg to 3.6 mmHg for DBP. In fact, given the within-group variability, these were not significant differences. Effects on other variables, such as left ventricular mass and ECG abnormalities, also failed to reveal important differences.

The Veteran's Administration Co-operative Study Group (VACSG) compared six agents with placebo: hydrochlorothiazide, atenolol, captopril, the centrally-acting sympatholytic clonidine, prazosin, and a modified-release formulation of diltiazem. The trial recruited nearly 1300 men, just under half of whom were black, who had DBP between 95 mmHg and 109 mmHg. Once again, all treatments were clearly superior to placebo, but in the VACSG study there were some apparent differences in efficacy. Overall, diltiazem was just the most effective in terms of blood pressure reduction, at least as regards DBP, and was effective in reducing DBP below 90 mmHg in 75% of treated patients. The other drugs produced response rates, by the above criterion, between 54% and 65%, while placebo produced responses in 33% of patients. Perhaps more importantly, the authors concluded that treatment had to be tailored to the individual patient (while recognizing that their data could not necessarily be extrapolated to women). Incidentally, they noted that captopril and atenolol, which tend to suppress renin levels, were more effective in younger than in older white men, while in blacks of all ages diltiazem produced the best response. This finding was consistent with the previously reported observation that black and older white hypertensives tend to have low or even suppressed renin levels and tend to respond in a more positive manner to drugs such as thiazides and calcium channel blockers that actually increase renin levels, but lower blood pressure by other mechanisms.

There is further support for this finding from a recent, much smaller study from Cambridge, in which there was clearly superior efficacy for monotherapy with ACE inhibitors and beta-blockers in younger men. In clinical practice, there is general consensus that monotherapy may achieve target blood pressures in 50-60% of patients at most, though published trials for individual drugs are generally more optimistic. Some of the recent major trials, discussed in the next chapter, have tilted the balance even further against single-drug therapy. It is also very important to remember that most antihypertensive drug side-effects are dose-related (Table 7), though this effect is not so clear with ACE inhibitors. Despite this, one should not lose sight of the importance of attempting to make a rational choice for initial therapy. The principal bases for this must be:

- On the positive side, there may be trial evidence that the drug is likely to be particularly effective in a given patient. Some of these considerations have been mentioned previously. There is very substantial evidence, for instance, for the efficacy of the thiazides in the elderly, as well as known ethnic differences in response. There are also concurrent diseases that can affect the choice of medication (Table 8).
- On the negative side, there may be compelling reasons why a drug should be avoided in specific patients (Table 8). Some issues still remain controversial, notably the role of dihydropyridine calcium channel blockers in diabetic hypertensives. Currently, the general view is that long-acting agents of this type are not harmful and may be beneficial, especially in terms of renoprotection and even more so when combined with angiotensin-converting enzyme inhibitors, but unfortunately the quality of much of the data is disappointing.

Table 7 *Some dose-related and unrelated adverse effects of antihypertensive drugs.*

Drug	Dose-related	Dose-unrelated
Thiazides	Hypokalaemia Dyslipidaemia Glucose intolerance Impotence	Gout*
Beta-blockers	Bradycardia† Cold extremities† Dyslipidaemia† Negative inotropy†	Bronchospasm* Nightmares*
Calcium channel blockers	Headaches, flushing Ankle oedema Bradycardia‡ Negative inotropy‡	
ACE inhibitors	Postural hypotension	Renal impairment in renovascular disease Angioedema Cough
Alpha blockers	Postural hypotension Sedation	
Sympatholoytics	Sedation Oedema	Dry mouth*

ACE: angiotensin converting enzyme.
* May occur at any clinically useful dose; † Note differences between subclasses of beta-blockers; ‡ For verapamil and diltiazem not dihydropyridines.

Targets and guidelines: how successful are we?

Given the greatly expanded range of therapies available, as well as the emphasis on individualized approaches to selecting medication, the above question is a very reasonable one. It is made more acute by the increasingly ambitious targets set by bodies such as the International and British Societies of Hypertension and the US Joint National Committee (Table 2). There are now

Table 8 *Indications and contraindications of major classes of antihypertensive drugs.*

	Indicated		Contraindicated	
	++	+	–	– –
Thiazides[*]	Elderly ISH	Heart failure	Dyslipidaemia	Gout
Beta-blockers	Angina Post-infarct	Heart failure[†] PVD Dyslipidaemia	Heart failure PVD[‡]	Heart block Asthma, COPD
CCBs (DHP)[§]	Elderly ISH	PVD Diabetes	–	Heart failure
CCBs (other)	Angina	Post-MI[**]	–	Heart block Heart failure
Alpha-blockers	BPH	Dyslipidaemia	Postural hypotension	Incontinence
ACE inhibitors	Heart failure LV dysfunction Diabetic nephropathy	Post-MI	–	Pregnancy Renovascular disease

contd.

Table 8 *Contd.*

	Indicated		Contraindicated	
	++	+	–	– –
AIIRAs	ACE inhibitor Cough	–	–	as ACE inhibitors
Sympatholytics[||]	–	Type 2 diabetes	–	–

ACE: angiotensin converting enzyme; AIIRA – angiotensin (AT_1) receptor antagonist; BPH: benign prostatic hypertrophy; CCB: calcium channel blocker; COPD: chronic obstructive pulmonary disease; DHP: dihydropyridine; ISH: isolated systolic hypertension; LV: left ventricular; MI: myocardial infarction; PVD: peripheral vascular disease.

[*] effects on lipids and uric acid less with indapamide;

[†] may be used under defined conditions in mild/moderate but not severe heart failure;

[‡] relevance in claudication uncertain, definitely contraindicated in Raynaud's phenomenon;

[§] long-acting drugs only;

[**] if patient not able to tolerate beta-blockers (particularly asthma, COPD);

[||] not discussed in current guidelines.

extensive data from many countries. The results are discouraging, to say the least. A recent US study of 800 hypertensive men with a mean age of around 65 years showed that 40% had blood pressure above 160/90 mmHg despite six or more clinic visits a year, in excellent centres, and over 75% had blood pressure higher than 140/90 mmHg. As might be expected, more intensive therapy, as judged by the frequency of increases in the number of drugs or their dose, was associated with better results. Results from a Spanish survey were somewhat worse, and data from the UK, Canada, Germany, and France were no better (although the most recent French data suggest that some 50% of hypertensive women and a third of hypertensive men have acceptable blood-pressure control). Although the now rather clichéd 'rule of halves' may no longer be wholly applicable, improvement is due mostly to better detection and greater awareness of hypertension: treatment is generally not more successful in those who are identified as hypertensive. Why not? Obviously there is no single answer, but the following issues are likely to be relevant:

- Clinicians are satisfied with modest improvements in blood pressure and fail to pursue targets, even when they claim otherwise: the 'something is better than nothing' approach. The Cardiomonitor study is particularly revealing in this respect: although 95% of patients and 76% of doctors thought hypertension was 'controlled', in fact BP was below 160/90 mmHg in only 37% of cases!
- The drug may not be the optimal choice from the outset, and additions or replacements may be similarly inappropriate.
- Secondary hypertension may not be recognized, and contributory problems such as obesity may not be successfully managed.
- Patients do not continue (or even may not start) treatment because of failure to understand the reasons for it, because of resistance to the idea of long-term drug therapy, because they cannot afford the cost of treatment or because of drug

side-effects. As an indication of the size of the problem, a large survey of hypertensive patients in general practices in the UK in 1995 showed that 40-50% of patients discontinued their initial medication within 6 months, irrespective of the class of drug involved, although more recent data on the angiotensin II receptor antagonists have been more positive. In most cases the drug was altered to one from another class, though one could not tell whether efficacy or side-effects was the stronger determinant in such a transition. About one-third of the cost of treating hypertension can be attributed to patients who switch or discontinue therapy.

Combination therapy in hypertension

Obviously, the present situation does not represent ideal or even acceptable blood pressure control, even though perfect control at a population level is unattainable. What can be done about it? As always in clinical medicine, communication between doctor and patient is vital, if not always as readily attainable as both would like. We must also try not to miss underlying causes of hypertension, though these may not always lead to 'cure' even if identified, and to take our own targets seriously (we all know how tempting it may be not to do so). In addition, clinicians can consider the following:

- Try to choose initial therapy rationally, taking into account the points already noted.
- Consider newly-introduced drugs, even though the information available may be rather sparse, but most definitely not at the expense of established agents for which evidence is more extensive.
- Consider combination therapy, 'free' combinations using two or more agents, or with fixed-dose formulations. In this context it is now well-known that in the Hypertension Optimal Treatment (HOT) Study and the United Kingdom Prospective Diabetes Study (UKPDS) about two-thirds of patients needed two or more drugs to attain blood pressures of around 140/85 mmHg.

The rational basis for combination therapy

What are we trying to gain from combination therapies in hypertension? The case for combination therapy has both a theoretical and a practical basis. Most antihypertensive drugs can be combined, and there are relatively few cases in which a particular combination is inappropriate or hazardous (Table 9). They may then:

- Complement each other in terms of *efficacy*, because of differing modes of action producing additive or occasionally synergistic effects.
- Counteract each other's *side-effects*, or
- Have *both* of these properties.

In several of the examples quoted below, drugs in combination are balancing out counter-regulatory systems that may tend to raise blood pressure in the presence of only one of the agents: for instance, thiazides and ACE inhibitors (Figure 7).

It must always be remembered that 'essential' hypertension is a heterogeneous condition, even if we do not have a very good understanding of the nature of the heterogeneity. In practical terms, therefore, we are looking for:

- Increased efficacy, with greater numbers of patients achieving target blood pressures.
- Certainly no more and preferably fewer side-effects and improved quality of life.
- Improved compliance because of fewer adverse effects, and, if possible
- Improved target organ protection
- Without significant extra cost, or even lowered cost(!)

Table 9 *Rational drug combinations.*

	Thiazides	Beta-blockers	CCBs (DHP)	CCBs (other)	Alpha-blockers	ACE I	AIIR	Sympatholytics
Thiazides	A	B	B, A	B, A	B	C	C	B
Beta-blockers	A	A	B	D	B	B	B	?
CCBs (DHP)	A	A	A	D	C	C	B	B
CCBs (other)	A	A	A	A	B	B	?	?
Alpha-blockers	A	A	A	A	A	B	?	D
ACE inhibitors	A	A	A	A	A	A	?	B
AIIRAs	A	A	A	A	A	A	A	?

ACE I: angiotensin converting enzyme inhibitor; AIIR: angiotensin (AT_1) receptor; AIIRA: angiotensin (AT_1) receptor antagonist; CCB: calcium channel blocker; DHP: dihydropyridine.

A: not applicable; B: rational; C: effective; D: not recommended; ?: data limited or absent.

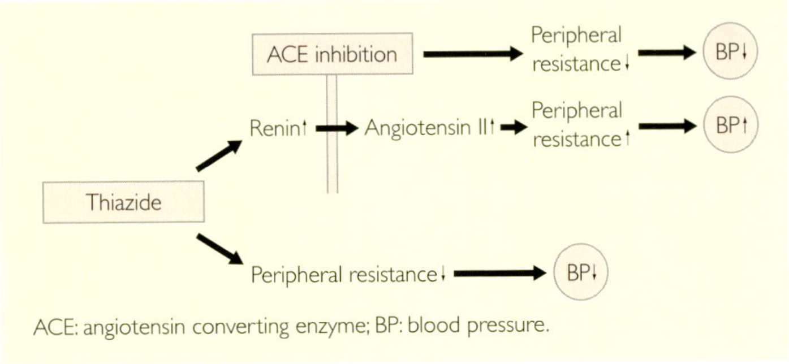

Figure 7 *Effect of drug combinations on counter-regulatory systems.*

Possible combinations — which are useful?

In fact, most combinations are useful. It will not be particularly helpful to consider all possible combinations, but the most widely-used ones are to be discussed here.

ACE inhibitors and thiazides, or thiazide-related diuretics

This is one of the best-established combinations, both as free combinations and in fixed-dose formulations. In fact, the latter are almost the most common fixed-dose combination antihypertensive products world-wide. There is a strong pharmacological case for this combination (Figure 7).

- Both drugs reduce peripheral resistance but by quite different mechanisms (in the case of thiazides, rather obscure ones).
- Thiazides activate the renin-angiotensin system while ACE inhibitors suppress the formation of angiotensin II, its principal product.

- ACE inhibitors will counteract thiazide-induced hypokalaemia, by reducing aldosterone secretion and probably also by the reduced direct effect of angiotensin II on renal tubules. They may also reduce hyperuricaemia caused by the thiazides.

- ACE inhibitors enhance the natriuretic action of the thiazides, though this probably does not have a major role in long-term blood pressure reduction. A particularly important role for this drug combination is in groups of hypertensive patients with low renin levels, notably Afro-Caribbeans. Similar considerations apply to the combination of angiotensin (AT_1) receptor antagonists with thiazides, and this combination has also become frequently used in the relatively short time that the receptor blockers have been available.

ACE inhibitors and dihydropyridine calcium channel blockers

These two types of drug are essentially peripheral vasodilators, but act by entirely different mechanisms. There are also other considerations that favour this combination:

- Dihydropyridines tend to activate both the sympathetic nervous system and the renin-angiotensin system, which can potentially blunt their antihypertensive effect: both these effects will be counteracted by ACE inhibition.

- Both drugs promote natriuresis.

- Dihydropyridine-induced ankle oedema seems to be diminished by ACE inhibitors.

- Both may protect renal function in diabetic hypertensives. It must be reiterated that short-acting dihydropyridines have no place at all in the acute or chronic management of hypertension.

ACE inhibitors and non-dihydropyridine calcium channel blockers

Most of the same points as above are relevant, although calcium channel blockers such as verapamil and diltiazem tend to cause much less sympathetic activation than the dihydropyridines, and in fact tend to reduce heart rate. They also cause less ankle oedema than the dihydropyridines.

Beta-blockers and dihydropyridine calcium channel blockers

This combination is a different situation, since the mode of action of the two drugs is really radically different. Beta-blockers do not generally reduce peripheral resistance, and sometimes the contrary occurs. There are several potential advantages:

- Beta-blockers reduce sympathetic activation associated with the calcium channel blockers.
- Beta-blockers block the increased renin release caused by vasodilatation. Calcium channel blockers counteract the vasoconstriction which may occur with most beta-blockers.

Beta-blockers and thiazides

This combination will be familiar to anyone accustomed to the stepped-care approach of the 1970s, when these were the principal classes of drugs available. Most clinical outcome data in hypertension have been obtained with one or both of these two classes of drugs. They also complement each other:

- Diuretics increase renin secretion, partly by promoting natriuresis and partly (probably) by vasodilatation.
- Beta-blockers inhibit renin secretion, as previously mentioned.

However, not all their interactions are favourable. In particular, both drugs may have dose-related adverse effects on the lipid profile, by increasing triglyceride levels and reducing concentrations of HDLs. This may promote atherogenesis, though the clinical relevance is unproven.

Calcium channel blockers (dihydropyridines) and alpha-blockers

This is another situation in which two different type of vasodilator are used together. Potentially, there could be increased postural hypotension but in practice this is rarely a problem. Neither class of drug produces adverse metabolic effects.

Do combinations work?

Given that one can make *theoretically* convincing cases for many specific combinations, it is reasonable to ask: how good is the evidence that they actually work? A short book such as this cannot comprehensively describe all outcomes of all possible combinations, even if these were available. In fact they are not, since relatively few have been tested rigorously in any case. This approach would require a factorial design to determine the optimal ratio of two drugs and to make a valid comparison with the individual components of the preparation.

The US Food and Drug Administration (FDA) has stipulated the following stringent requirements for fixed-dose combinations, which are worth bearing in mind for combinations in general: (a) the combination should be more effective than the sum of its components; (b) the combined product must be at least as safe as its component parts; (c) the risk to benefit ratio should be better than for either component alone. These are very ambitious targets, but they have given added impetus for careful studies of this issue. In practice, most studies have included a thiazide or thiazide-like diuretic, so it may be helpful to divide the data broadly into diuretic and non-diuretic studies.

Diuretic-based combinations

The concept of a low or very low dose of diuretic added to another drug has recently attracted increasing interest. It is now generally accepted that the inclusion of these drugs will almost always enhance the efficacy of any combination therapy. In the USA the combination of hydrochlorothiazide at a dose of just 6.25 mg is available in combination with the relatively cardio-selective beta-blocker bisoprolol (2.5 mg, 5 mg and 10 mg daily) and has been approved for once-daily dosage in the initial treatment of hypertension. The effects on blood pressure of a factorial study are shown in Table 10. With the 6.25/10 combination, about two-thirds of moderately hypertensive patients have DBP reduced to 90 mmHg or less. Although there may be somewhat greater efficacy with 25 mg hydrochlorothiazide, this would be at the expense of more adverse effects.

Far more combinations involve a thiazide diuretic and an ACE inhibitor. In most publications the thiazide used is hydrochlorothiazide, typically at a dose of 12.5-25 mg, though at higher doses in some of the earlier studies. For instance, among many reports:

- Patients with moderate hypertension were randomly assigned to enalapril 10 mg bd, hydrochlorothiazide 25 mg bd, or a combination of the two. Only 7% of patients taking enalapril alone

Table 10 *Antihypertensive effects of various doses of bisoprolol and hydrochlorothiazide in combination.*

		Bisoprolol (mg)		
		0	10	20
	0	–	-4.6	-7.1
HCTZ (mg)	2.5	-2.6	-7.0	-9.6
	5	-4.6	-9.1	-11.6

HCTZ = hydrochlorothiazide.
Figures are placebo-corrected changes in diastolic blood pressure (mmHg). Adapted from Frishman et al, 1994.

achieved DBP <90 mmHg, as did only 15% of those on thiazide alone, compared to 80% of those taking both.

- In a much larger trial, patients were given lisinopril (20-80 mg daily, hydrochlorothiazide (12.5-50 mg daily) or combination therapy with both (three combinations over the same dose range for each drug). Doses were titrated to achieve DBP <90mm Hg. Mean SBP/DBP reductions for the three groups were: 16.6/12.5; 10.4/6.8 and 23.9/18.2.
- Patients were randomly assigned to perindopril >4 mg daily, hydrochlorothiazide 25 mg daily, or both. Treatment with either single drug produce similar falls in SBP/DBP (11/7 mmHg), while in combination the effect was additive (24.5/12.6 mmHg).

Recently, a new combination has been introduced, incorporating the long-acting ACE inhibitor perindopril at a dose of 2 mg and the non-thiazide diuretic indapamide at a dose of 0.625 mg. These are, respectively, one half and one quarter of the usual maintenance doses of these drugs in their standard formulations. The combined preparation is designed to harmonize the pharmacokinetic profiles of its two components and the trough-peak ratio is about 0.6, which can be considered acceptable. The results of somewhat incomplete dose-finding studies are summarized in Table 11, although in further efficacy studies in more than 380 patients the reduction in blood pressure in patients with mild-to-moderate hypertension after 12 weeks' treatment was higher at 10.7/6.0 mmHg, corrected for placebo. This finding gave a responder rate of 81% compared with 49% for placebo (DBP ≤90 mmHg); or reductions of diastolic blood pressure by at least 10 mmHg and systolic pressure by 10 mmHg, or 20 mmHg in the case of ISH. Apart from a slight increase in cough tolerability was very good, with negligible effects on serum biochemical parameters such as potassium, uric acid and glucose.

Table 11 *Antihypertensive effects of various doses of perindopril and indapamide in combination.*

		Perindopril (mg)			
		0	2	4	8
	0	–	–	-5.4	–
Indapamide (mg)	0.625	–	-4.1	-6.2	–
	1.25	-3.9	-4.4	-7.5	-6.7
	2.5	–	–	-9.2	-9.8

Figures are placebo-corrected changes in diastolic blood pressure (mmHg).
Adapted from Myers et al, 2000.

Non-diuretic based combinations

Although these combinations are considerably less common, interest in them has been increasing recently. In the USA the ACE inhibitor/calcium channel blocker combination of benazepril and amlodipine has been extensively studied, as part of the development of a combined product (Table 12). The 2.5/10 mg combination produces a greater response than the sum of its components, and the 5/20 combination is approximately additive. A recent study compared the dihydropyridine felodipine 10 mg daily with the following:

Table 12 *Antihypertensive effects of various doses of benazepril and amlodipine in combination.*

		Benazepril (mg)		
		0	10	20
	0	–	-2.4	-8.8
Amlodipine (mg)	2.5	-6.8	-13.4	-9.8
	5	-12.4	-11.2	-20.2

Figures are placebo-corrected changes in diastolic blood pressure (mmHg).
After Weir, 1998.

- felodipine 5 mg combined with enalapril 5 mg daily
- benazepril 10 mg/amlodipine 5 mg daily.

This followed a minimum period with felodipine 5 mg daily. Only 14% of patients achieved DBP ≤ 90 mmHg on the latter dose. After randomization, reductions in clinic BP were: for felodipine 14.9/8.3 mmHg; for felodipine/enalapril 13.6/7.5 mmHg; and for benazepril/amlodipine 18.6/10.7 mmHg. This is an unusual trial design but nonetheless it does suggest at least equivalence for low-dose combinations compared with titration of single drugs.

A combined formulation of trandolapril and verapamil is now also available. A large factorial study with verapamil modified-release (120 mg or 180 mg daily), trandolapril (0.5, 1.0 or 2.0 mg daily), and all combinations of these, showed a clear advantage for the combinations (Table 13). This finding was particularly marked for verapamil 180 mmHg with trandolapril 0.5 mg or 1.0 mg.

Felodipine and modified-release metoprolol (a relatively cardioselective beta-blocker) have also been studied both individually and in combination. The doses were felodipine 5-10 mg daily, metoprolol 50-100 mg daily or felodipine plus metoprolol 5/50-10/100 mg daily. Blood pressure control, as judged by DBP

Table 13 *Antihypertensive effects of various doses of verapamil SR and trandolapril in combination.*

		Verapamil SR (mg)		
		0	120	180
	0	–	-11.2	-8.9
Trandolapril (mg)	0.5	-10.7	-14.4	-14.1
	1.0	-10.8	-14.0	-16.0
	2.0	-13.9	-15.1	-15.2

Figures are placebo-corrected changes in diastolic blood pressure (mmHg).
After Scholze et al, 1998.

≤ 90 mmHg, was achieved in 45% of patients on felodipine, in 40% of those on metoprolol, and in 71% of those taking the combination of the two.

The efficacy of combinations: an overview

It is very difficult to compare trials of combination therapy, for obvious reasons. There is no overall co-ordination of international trial design and, as for any meta-analysis, eventually one resorts to setting some minimum standards for comparability. A recent analysis assembled data from 17 double-blind randomized studies with a factorial design, involving pair-wise combinations of four major classes of antihypertensive drugs and nearly 3 000 patients. The results are summarised in Table 14. In these studies, the results are compatible with an additive effect of the drugs in each pair and nothing more. These results seem to caution against expecting spectacular results from combination therapy, but earlier comments will already have indicated that such results should not be anticipated in any case.

Table 14 *Drug combinations and blood pressure lowering. Reproduced with kind permission of Messerli and Michalewicz (1997).*

	A	B	C	D
B	–	–	–	104 (12, 416)
C	101 (23, 1503)	–	–	97 (17, 351)
D	96 (18, 737)	104 (12, 416)	97 (17, 351)	–

A: ACE inhibitors; B: beta-blockers; C: calcium channel blockers; D: diuretics. Figures are percentage decreases compared to that predicted from additive effects of the two drugs. Figures in parentheses are the numbers of studies analysed, and total numbers of patients.

Prospects for combination therapy

Are fixed-dose combinations still controversial?

It is inevitable that individualized combinations will evolve during the course of the management of individual hypertensive patients: as we have seen, most patients will need such combinations for satisfactory control. However, there is still disagreement on the role of fixed-dose combinations, particularly as a basis for initial therapy. Such combinations have been discouraged in the past, especially in the UK, and particularly by academic clinical pharmacologists such as myself. Some controversy still remains but the fixed-dose concept has become more widely acceptable, particularly as regards low-dose combinations. Recent guidelines, including those of the US Joint National Committee and the British Hypertension Society, agree that these preparations are appropriate at least in some circumstances. Obviously, the combination should be safe and rational one in the first place. The following advantages may follow, in addition to these seen with combination therapy in general:

- Reduced numbers of tablets, with potentially improved adherence by patients.
- Depending on the national funding system and the manufacturers' pricing structure, reduced costs to the patients, the funding authorities, or both.

- The use of doses of drugs that may be lower than those available individually, especially in the case of thiazide diuretics.

However, possible disadvantages cannot be totally ignored:

- Reduced flexibility in the dosage of individual components.
- Discrepancies in the pharmacokinetics of the component drugs.
- The danger that prescribers may not bear in mind exactly what the combination contains, especially as regards the contraindications of the individual components.

The first of these issues is undoubtedly a genuine problem. Its effect can be reduced by producing several different combined formulations, but this may be confusing and probably expensive. A simpler approach is to recognize that these preparations should be used only over a narrow dose range, usually only one or two tablets. It is obviously desirable that chosen doses are based on careful investigations of the possible different combinations, as described above. The second issue can be foreseen and avoided by the use of appropriate formulations: examples already quoted include extended-release formulations of indapamide and metoprolol, which were combined with intrinsically long-acting drugs (perindopril and felodipine). The third issue is largely a matter of education: as such it can be minimized but will be difficult if not impossible to avoid altogether.

New approaches

New combinations — present and future

We are not in the happy position of saying that there are enough drugs to treat hypertension, even though so many already exist. Although one would suppose that all combinations have been tried, some will probably be exploited further. One of these is the combination of ACE inhibitors with AT_1 antagonists. This combination may seem strange but as Figure 8

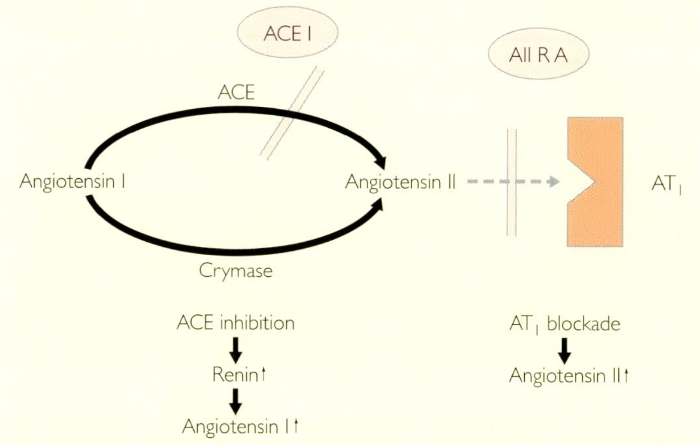

ACE: angiotensin converting enzyme; ACE I: angiotensin converting enzyme inhibitor; AIIRA: angiotensin (AI$_1$) receptor antagonist.

Figure 8 *New combinations: ACE inhibitors with AT$_1$ antagonists.*

shows it is in fact quite rational. So far only very limited evidence exists for the efficacy of this combination, but it is being investigated further. Further new classes of antihypertensive drugs are now in development. One of these, the vasopeptidase inhibitors, will almost certainly have been launched by the time this book is published. These compounds have dual properties: they are ACE inhibitors and they also inhibit the enzyme neutral endopeptidase, thereby increasing levels of the natriuretic peptides. The efficacy of these agents is very promising and it remains to be seen which other drugs will be most suitable for combinations — though it is possible that these will be less frequently needed. Obviously, ACE inhibitors will not be relevant, but the angiotensin receptor antagonists may be suitable, as may most of the other drug classes. Rather further from clinical use are the endothelin receptor antagonists, which block the action of this very potent vasoconstrictor. In principle, almost any potential combination may prove useful if and when these drugs reach clinicians.

Not just what, but also when?

Blood pressure follows a diurnal rhythm in all people with normal blood pressure and in most hypertensives. So does the incidence of cardiovascular events, which shows a marked rise on getting up in the morning associated with rises in blood pressure and heart rate (Figure 9). The control of blood pressure should try to take account of these facts:

- Adequate control should be maintained over the full 24 hours, since there is evidence that less comprehensive control is associated with reduced benefit from treatment.
- The morning surge in blood pressure should be avoided or minimized.

The first of these objectives has received much greater attention than the second. Almost all treatment strategies are directed at once-daily dosing with adequate control throughout the day, usu-

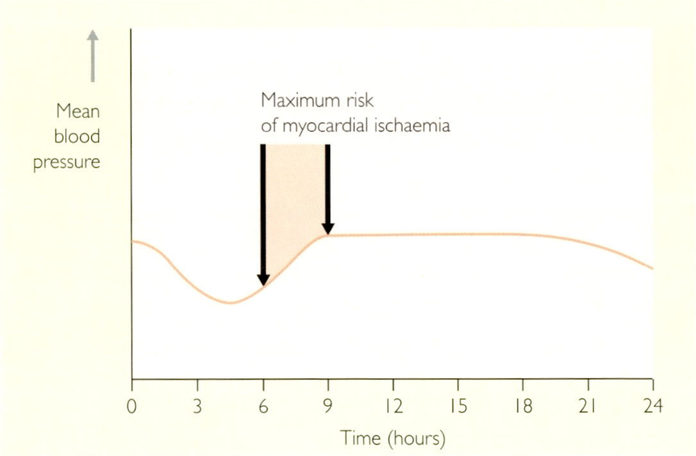

Figure 9 *Normal diurnal blood pressure rhythm.*

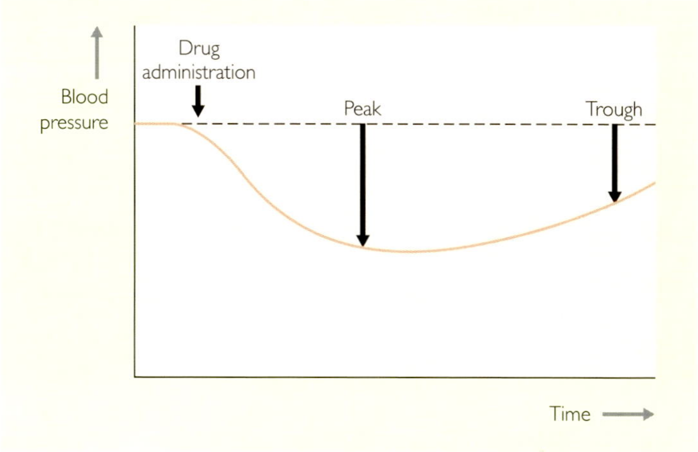

Figure 10 *Characteristic trough-peak ratio of once-daily dosing treatments.*

ally characterized by the trough-peak ratio (Figure 10). The FDA has set a threshold of 0.5 for this ratio if a drug is to be described as a once-daily drug, but most clinicians would regard that threshold as inadequate and aim for a value of at least 0.7. The whole concept of the trough-peak ratio has been extensively criticized, but it remains by far the most widely recognized single figure for describing the duration of action of antihypertensive drugs. Alternative approaches, such as the smoothness index, await large-scale validation. The problem of the early-morning rise in blood pressure is naturally linked, but deserves particular emphasis because of the potential clinical consequences. There are three broad approaches:

- Changing the formulations.
- Changing the timing of monotherapy.
- Using drugs in combination, administered at different times.

There has been interest in chronotherapeutics, which refers to the development of delivery systems that allow drug release not only over an extended period but also at specific times in each 24-hour cycle. This process has been explored in other therapeutic areas, such as cancer chemotherapy, as well as in hypertension.

Several delivery systems have been developed for the treatment of hypertension, mostly using verapamil as the therapeutic agent, which are designed to produce maximum plasma levels of drug between 0600 hours and 1200 hours. However, these formulations do not seem to have entered clinical practice, though whether for clinical or commercial reasons is unclear. Several studies have compared the efficacy of evening drug administration with the conventional practice of taking the drugs at or after breakfast. There are two potential problems with evening administration. First, blood pressure may fall too much at a time when it is in any case at its lowest, between 0000 hours and 0300 hours. Though this is unlikely to be noticed by the patient, it could potentially lead to hypoperfusion in already-compromised vascular beds, especially in the heart and brain. Second, and probably more importantly, blood pressure control may be lost during the late morning and afternoon. Data on this point are contradictory, for instance with discrepant results from the same authors comparing the ACE inhibitors benazepril and quinapril. Overall, it seems unlikely that monotherapy would be a satisfactory solution.

The final and most practicable approach is, once again, combination therapy. Some drugs (for instance doxazosin) may blunt the morning rise when taken in the evening but by themselves will not provide adequate 24-hour blood pressure control. They can then be combined with other agents which may be longer-acting and would be taken as usual in the morning. It would be rational to use a drug such as doxazosin or a sympatholytic in the evening since they act indirectly or directly on the sympathetic nervous system, which is directly involved in the morning arousal response. In addition, this type of drug can cause sedation, which might be a positive advantage at night, but a nuisance during the day. On the negative side, one loses the advantage of once-daily dosing.

Summary and questions

Attitudes to the treatment of hypertension have changed and are changing. The outcome of these changes will be greater demands on the clinician and perhaps also on the patient, but it will be some years before we know whether they will result in long-term reductions in morbidity and mortality. The following is a summary of a personal, perhaps not too controversial, view:

- We need to aim at lower targets for our hypertensive patients: about 140/85 mmHg and less in diabetics.
- This will only be achievable by monotherapy in only a minority of patients.
- Most of the major classes of antihypertensives can be effectively and safely used in combination.
- Low-dose combination therapy can and should be considered as an early alternative to escalating the dose in monotherapy.
- In addition to greater efficacy, this may also result in fewer side-effects.
- Fixed low-dose combinations are an acceptable treatment option, including initial therapy, provided that there is adequate clinical evidence for the particular formulation.
- Combination therapy given more than once daily may be useful in smoothing 24-hour blood pressure control and especially in buffering early-morning peaks of blood pressure.
- Combination therapy will almost always be enhanced by inclusion of low-dose or very-low-dose thiazides.

Aside from the question of long-term clinical outcomes there are other outstanding issues. One important and closely-related question concerns the issue of target organ protection: are some combinations particularly beneficial independent of blood pressure reduction? The calcium-channel-blocker controversy in diabetes has been mentioned earlier, but for most other combinations this amount of evidence is not available.

There are two further points to consider, though both are unlikely to be fully investigated because of the complexity of the questions. Does the order in which drugs are given in combination matter? In other words, is A then B the same as B then A? Very limited evidence suggests that it may not be in some cases. What are the data for triple or even quadruple therapy? Very scanty. A significant minority of patients will receive multiple therapy, not just double therapy, and we do not have any systematic data on this issue.

What is the most appropriate conclusion at the end of this book? A simple one: the important thing is to lower blood pressure successfully: the ends justify the means! In most cases, combination therapy will be the means.

Further reading

Key Books

Beevers DG, MacGregor GA. *Hypertension in Practice*, 3rd edn. London: Martin Dunitz, 1999.

Kaplan NM, *Clinical Hypertension*, 7th edn. Baltimore: Williams & Wilkins, 1998.

Opie LH, Messerli FH, eds. *Combination Drug Therapy for Hypertension*. New York: Authors Publishing House/Lippincott-Raven, 1997.

The problem of hypertension

Birkett NJ. The effect of alternative criteria for hypertension on estimates of prevalence and control. *J Hypertens* 1997;**15**:237–22.

Burt VL, Whelton P, Roccella EJ et al. Prevalence of hypertension in the US adult population. Results from the Third National Health and Nutrition Examination Survey, 1988–1991. *J Hypertens* 1995;**25**:305–13.

Carretero OA, Oparil S. Essential hypertension: part I: definition and etiology. *Circulation* 2000;**101**:329–35.

Guidelines Subcommittee. 1999 World Health Organization – International Society of Hypertension Guidelines for the Management of Hypertension. *J Hypertens* 1999;**17**:151–83.

Kannel VB. Blood pressure as a cardiovascular risk factor. *JAMA* 1996;**275**:1571–5.

McInnes GT, Semple PF. Hypertension: investigation, assessment and diagnosis. *Br Med Bull* 1994;**50**:443–59.

Rahn KH, Brenbrock M, Hausberg M. The sympathetic nervous system in the pathogenesis of hypertension. *J Hypertens* 1999;**17**(suppl 3):S11–14.

Ram CV. Renovascular hypertension. *Curr Opin Nephrol Hypertens* 1997;**6**:575–9.

Ramsay LE, Williams B, Johnston GD et al. Guidelines for management of hypertension: report of the third working party of the British Hypertension Society. *J Hum Hypertens* 1999;**13**:569–92.

Sixth Report of the Joint National Committee on Prevention, Detection and Evaluation and Treatment of High Blood Pressure. *Arch Int Med* 1997;**157**:2413–46.

Werbel SS, Ober KP. Pheochromocytoma. Update on diagnosis, localization, and management. *Med Clin North Am* 1995;**79**:131–53.

Young WF Jr. Primary aldosteronism: a common and curable form of hypertension. *Cardiol Rev* 1999;**7**:207–14.

The treatment of hypertension

Anderson NB, Myers HF, Pickering T, Jackson JS. Hypertension in blacks: psychosocial and biological perspectives. *J Hypertens* 1989;**7**:161–72.

Appel LJ. Nonpharmacologic therapies that reduce blood pressure: a fresh perspective. *Clin Cardiol* 1999;**22**:111, 1–5.

Berlowitz DR, Ash AS, Hickey EC et al. Inadequate management of blood pressure in a hypertensive population. *N Engl J Med* 1998;**339**:1957–63.

Chokalingam A, Fodor JG. Treatment of raised blood pressure in the population: the Canadian experience. *Am J Hypertens* 1998;**11**:747–9.

Colhoun HM, Dong W, Poulter NR. Blood pressure screening, management and control in England: results from the health survey for England 1994. *J Hypertens* 1998;**16**:747–52.

Cutler JA, Follmann D, Allender PS. Randomized trials of sodium reduction: an overview. *Am J Clin Nutr* 1997;**65**(suppl 2):643S–651S.

Dahlof B, Jonsson L, Borgholst O et al. Improved antihypertensive efficacy of the felodipine-metoprolol extended-release tablet compared with each drug alone. *Blood Press* 1993;**1**(suppl):37–45.

Dickerson JE, Hingorani AD, Ashby MJ et al. Optimisation of antihypertensive treatment by crossover rotation of four major classes. *Lancet* 1999;**353**:2008–13.

Faulhaber H-D, Luft FC. Treatment of high blood pressure in Germany. *Am J Hypertens* 1998;**11**:750–3.

Hosie J, Wiklund I. Managing hypertension in general practice: can we do better? *J Hum Hypertens* 1995;**9**(suppl 2):S15–S18.

Hughes D, McGuire A. The direct costs to the NHS of discontinuing and switching prescriptions for hypertension. *J Hum Hypertens* 1998;**12**:533–7.
Jones JK, Gorkin L, Lian JF et al. Discontinuation of and changes in treatment after start of new courses of antihypertensive drugs: a study of the United Kingdom population. *BMJ* 1995;**3119**:293–5.
Pardell H, Tresseras R, Armario P, Hernandez R. Actions implemented to improve hypertension control in Spain. *Am J Hypertens* 1998;**1**:763–5.
Poggi L, Chamontin B, Lang T et al. An attempt to improve blood pressure control in the French population. Information and outcome awareness at the general practitioner level. *Am J Hypertens* 1998;**11**:905–8.
Scholze J, Zilles P, Compagnone D. Verapamil SR and trandolapril combination therapy in hypertension – a clinical trial of factorial design. *Br J Clin Pharmacol* 1998;**45**:491–5.
Sheinfeld GR, Bakris GL. Benefits of combination angiotensin-converting enzyme inhibitor and calcium antagonist therapy for diabetic patients. *Am J Hypertens* 1999;**12**:80S–85S.
Trials of Hypertension Prevention Collaboration Research Group. The effects of nonpharmacologic interventions of blood pressure of persons with high normal levels: results of the Trials of Hypertension Prevention, Phase I. *JAMA* 1992;**267**:1213–20.

Combination therapy in hypertension

Abernethy DR. Pharmacological properties of combination therapies for hypertension. *Am J Hypertens* 1997;**10**:13S–16S.
Aksoyek K, Ozer N, Aytemir K et al. Verapamil SR and trandolapril combination therapy is safe and effective in hypertensive patients with metabolic disorders. *Int J Clin Pract* 2001;**55**:5–9.
Ambrosioni E. Pharmacoeconomics of hypertension management: the place of combination therapy. *Pharmacoeconomics* 2001;**19**:337–47.
Brown CL, Backhouse CI, Grippat JC, Santoni JP. The effect of perindopril and hydrochlorothiazide alone and in combination on blood pressure and the renin-angiotensin system in hypertensive subjects. *Eur J Clin Pharmacol* 1990;**39**:327–32.
Frishman WH, Goldberger J, Sherman D. Enalapril, hydrochlorothiazide, and combination therapy in patients with moderate hypertension. *J Clin Hypertens* 1987;**3**:520–7.

Frishman WH, Bryzinski BS, Coulson LR et al. A multifactorial trial design to assess combination therapy in hypertension. Treatment with bisoprolol and hydrochlorothiazide. *Arch Intern Med* 1994;**154**:1461–8.

Hansson L, Zanchetti A, Carruthers SG et al. Effects of intensive blood-pressure lowering and low-dose aspirin in patients with hypertension: principal results of the Hypertension Optimal Treatment (HOT) randomised trial. HOT Study Group. *Lancet* 1998;**351**:1755–62.

Kaplan NM. Low-dose combination therapy: the rationalization for an ACE inhibitor and a calcium channel blocker in higher risk patients. *Am J Hypertens* 2001;**14**:8S–11S.

McLellan KJ, Markham A. Perindopril 2 mg/Indapamide 0.625 mg. Fixed low-dose combination. *Drugs* 1999;**58**:297–302.

Messerli FH, Oparil S, Feng Z. Comparison of efficacy and side-effects of combination therapy of angiotensin-converting enzyme inhibitor (benazepril) with calcium antagonist (either nifedipine or amlodipine) versus high-dose calcium antagonist monotherapy for systemic hypertension. *Am J Cardiol* 2000;**86**:1182–7.

Messerli FH. Combinations in the treatment of hypertension: ACE inhibitors and calcium antagonists. *Am J Hypertens* 1999;**12**:86S–90S.

Messerli FH, Michaelwicz L. Cardiac effects of combination therapy. *Am J Hypertens*. 1997;**10**:146S–152S.

Moser M, Black HR. The role of combination therapy in the treatment of hypertension. *Am J Hypertens* 1998;**11**:73S–78S.

Myers MG, Asmar R, Leenen FH, Safar M. Fixed low-dose combination therapy in hypertension – a dose response study of perindopril and indapamide. *J Hypertens* 2000;**18**:317–25.

Neutel JM. Low-dose antihypertensive combination therapy: its rationale and role in cardiovascular risk management. *Am J Hypertens* 1999;**12**:73S–79S.

Neutel JM, Smith DH, Weber MA. Low-dose combination therapy: an important first line treatment in the management of hypertension. *Am J Hypertens* 2001;**14**:286–92.

Neutel JM, Smith DHG, Weber MA. Low dose combination therapy vs. high dose monotherapy in the management of hypertension. *J Clin Hypertens* 1999;**1**:179–86.

Opie LH. Principles of combination therapy for hypertension: what we learn from the HOT and other studies – a personal point of view. *Cardiovasc Drugs Ther* 1998;**12**:425–9.

Pool JL, Gennari J, Goldstein R et al. Controlled multicenter study of the antihypertensive effects of Lisinopril, hydrochlorothiazide, and lisinopril plus hydrochlorothiazide in the treatment of 394 patients with mild to moderate hypertension. *J Cardiovasc Pharmacol* 1987;**9**(suppl 3): S36-42.

Ruzicka M, Leenen FH. Monotherapy versus combination therapy as first line treatment of uncomplicated arterial hypertension. *Drugs* 2001;**61**:943–54.

Scholze J, Zilles P, Compagnone D. Verapamil SR and trandolapril combination therapy in hypertension – a clinical trial of factorial design. German Hypertension Study Group. *Br J Clin Pharmacol* 1998;**45**:491–5.

UK Prospective Diabetes Study Group. Tight blood pressure control and risk of macrovascular and microvascular complications in type 2 diabetes: UKPDS 38. *BMJ* 1998;**317**:703–13.

Prospects for combination therapy

Anwar YA, White WB. Chronotherapeutics for cardiovascular disease. *Drugs* 1998;**55**:631–43.

Epstein M, Bakris G. Newer approaches to antihypertensive therapy. Use of fixed-dose combination therapy. *Arch Intern Med* 1996;**156**:1969–78.

Hilleman DE, Ryschon KL, Mohiuddin SM, Wurdeman RL. Fixed-dose combination vs monotherapy in hypertension: a meta-analysis evaluation. *J Hum Hypertens* 1999;**13**:477–83.

Johnstone MT, Mittelman M, Tofler G, Muller JE. The pathophysiology of the onset of morning cardiovascular events. *Am J Hypertens* 1996;**9**:22S–28S.

Materson BJ, Reda DJ, Williams D. Lessons from combination therapy in Veterans Affairs Studies. Department of Veterans Affairs Cooperative Study Group on antihypertensive agents. *Am J Hypertens* 1996;**9**:187S–191S.

Meredith PA. How to evaluate the duration of blood pressure control: the trough:peak ratio and 24-hour monitoring. *J Cardiovasc Pharmacol* 1998;**31**(suppl 2):S17–21.

Morgan T, Anderson A. How important is 24-hour control of blood pressure? *Drug Saf* 1996;**15**:243–8.

Morgan T, Anderson A, Jones E. The effect of 24h blood pressure control of an angiotensin converting enzyme inhibitor (perindopril) administered in the morning or at night. *J Hypertens* 1997;**15**:205–11.

Neutel JM, Smith DHG. The circadian pattern of blood pressure: cardiovascular risk and therapeutic opportunities. *Curr Opin Nephrol Hypertens* 1997;**6**:235–6.

Neutel JM, Smith DHG. The role of low-dose combination therapy in the management of hypertension: an alternative approach. *Hosp Med* 1998;**34**:35–43.

Palatini P, Racoppa A, Raule G et al. Effect of timing of administration on the plasma ACE inhibitory activity and the antihypertensive effect of quinapril. *Clin Pharmacol Ther* 1992;**52**:378–83.

Palatini P, Mos L, Motolese M et al. Effect of evening versus morning benazepril on 24-hour blood pressure: a comparative study with continuous intraarterial monitoring. *Int J Clin Pharamcol Ther Toxicol* 1993;**6**:295–300.

Parali G, Omboni S, Rizzoni D et al. The smoothness index: a new, reproducible and clinically relevant measure of the homogeneity of the blood pressure reduction with treatment for hypertension. *J Hypertens* 1998;**16**:1685–91.

Waeber B, Brunner HR. Combination antihypertensive therapy: does it have a role in rational therapy? *Am J Hypertens* 1997;**10**:131S–137S.

Weir MR. The rationale for combination versus single-entity therapy in hypertension. *Am J Hypertens* 1998;**11**:163S–169S.

White WB. A chronotherapeutic approach to the management of hypertension. *Am J Hypertens* 1996;**9**:29S–33S.

Index